Liver and Gallbladder Health

How to Prevent and Reverse Fatty Liver and Diet with or without a Gallbladder

By S.W. Livingston

Text Copyright © 2019 S.W. Livingston

All Rights Reserved

No part of this book may be reproduced
in any way without the written
permission of the author.

Disclaimer:
The views expressed within this book are those of the author alone. The information contained within this book is based on the opinions, experiences, and observations of the author and is provided "AS-IS". No warranties of any kind are made. Neither the author nor publisher are engaged in rendering professional services of any kind. Neither the author nor publisher will assume liability or responsibility for any loss or damage related directly or indirectly to the information contained within this book.

The author has attempted to be as accurate as possible with the information contained within this book. Neither the author nor publisher will assume responsibility or liability for any errors, omissions, inconsistencies, or inaccuracies.

Table of Contents

Introduction..
Why it's so Important to Have a Healthy Liver...
    Toxin Removal...
    Food Digestion..
    Protein and Enzyme Building...
Possible Warning Signs of an Unhealthy Liver..
    How to Keep Track of Symptoms...
Possible Causes of an Unhealthy Liver...
Gallstones...
    Symptoms...
    Causes...
    Risks..
Fatty Liver..
    Alcohol Related...
    Nonalcoholic Related..
    Risks..
    Diagnosis..
    What to Expect..
How to Relieve Liver and Gallbladder Pain Naturally......................................
How to Eliminate Gallstones or Prevent them from Occurring.......................
How to Reverse Fatty Liver..
How to Diet After Gallbladder Removal..
Closing..

Introduction

Since the liver has a very important role in the human anatomy, it is certainly essential for overall health.

Located under the ribs on the right side, it is one of the largest organs in the body, approximately the size of a football.

Here are some of the things the liver is responsible for:

- **Neutralizing and removing toxins**
- **Processing digested food**
- **Building proteins and enzymes**

Liver problems can interfere with these functions, so it's crucial to keep this organ healthy, especially since there is currently no known device that is able to effectively mimic all the functions of the liver.

The gallbladder, which is responsible for storing bile, is a pear-shaped organ that is located on the underside of the liver. Although it's not as important as the liver, it can still cause problems if it is not taken care of.

Whether you have gallstones, or have had your gallbladder removed and are wondering how you should diet, this book can help.

This book will teach you how to have a healthy liver and gallbladder.

It will cover:

- **Why it's so important to have a healthy liver**
- **Possible warning signs of an unhealthy liver**
- **Possible causes of an unhealthy liver**
- **How to relieve liver and gallbladder pain naturally**
- **How to eliminate gallstones or prevent them from occurring**
- **How to reverse fatty liver**
- **How to diet after gallbladder removal**
- **and plenty more**

Why it's so Important to Have a Healthy Liver

In order to understand and appreciate why it is so important to have a healthy liver, it is necessary to understand what the liver's primary functions are.

Although the Introduction chapter listed it's primary functions, this chapter will go into detail about those functions.

Note: This is not an exhaustive list, as the liver has other functions. The functions covered in this chapter are simply the functions in which the liver is primarily responsible for.

Toxin Removal

There are multiple ways toxins can get into the bloodstream, such as when:

- Ingesting something poisonous
- The body itself produces toxins to help break down protein

The liver essentially acts as a filter. Nutrients and chemicals that are consumed will pass through the liver.

From there, the liver takes the helpful substances that it needs and stores them.

Anything that is harmful or not needed will get passed on or converted into nonthreatening substances.

Aside from nutrients from food, medication and alcohol also stop by the liver while passing through the body.

Although medication and alcohol in small doses can be helpful, they are still considered toxic to an extent and must be filtered out by the liver, along with other toxins.

Food Digestion

The liver produces bile, which is a liquid that is used for the process of digestion. Bile emulsifies fats and aids in the absorption of vitamin K.

After the bile gets produced by the liver, it gets stored in the gallbladder. From there, it gets secreted into the small intestine.

The liver processes nutrients that have been absorbed by the small intestine.

Since the digestion system is responsible for converting food into energy, the liver contributes to providing the body with energy.

Protein and Enzyme Building

The liver largely contributes to the synthesis of amino acids, which are the building blocks of protein.

The liver is also largely responsible for making a protein hormone called *insulin-like growth factor 1*, which allows children to grow and has an anabolic effect on people in their adulthood.

Most of the body's lipoproteins are synthesized in the liver.

Possible Warning Signs of an Unhealthy Liver

Some signs of liver damage are more subtle than others, which is why it is important to pay attention to even the small details.

Abdominal Pain

This is one of the more obvious ones. If the abdominal region hurts, particularly where the liver is located, it can be a sign is either struggling with inflammation or damage.

The pain might go away but then return at a later time.

Yellowing of the eyes

A malfunctioning liver can cause a certain compound that causes jaundice to accumulate in the bloodstream.

Blemishes on face

Brownish pigmentation can occur on the face when the liver is not functioning optimally. When the liver is not functioning well, it can cause an enzyme to produce extra skin pigmentation.

Reddening of the palms

Another sign of liver damage is when the palms of the hands turn red. This redness can be accompanied by a burning or itching sensation.

Sluggishness and lack of focus

As stated in an earlier chapter, the liver plays a role in digestion, and since the digestion system is responsible for converting food into energy, the liver contributes to providing the body with energy.

Therefore, when the liver is not functioning correctly, it can cause a person to experience a lack of energy.

This lack of energy can interfere with a person's ability to focus.

Bleeding too easily

Since proteins can be used to cause blood clots, and since the liver is largely responsible for building those proteins, bleeding or bruising too easily can be a sign of a compromised liver.

Itchiness of skin

A malfunctioning liver can allow bile to get released into the bloodstream. The bile running through the bloodstream can cause the skin to itch.

How to Keep Track of Symptoms

Certain symptoms associated with an unhealthy liver can mimic other illnesses. For this reason, it can be beneficial to keep track of any symptoms you may be experiencing.

You can keep track of your symptoms by:

- **Writing your symptoms down in a journal**
- **Documenting the date in which you started noticing the symptoms**
- **Monitoring if certain food products or activities make the symptoms better or worse**
- **Taking pictures of any visibly noticeable symptoms, such as a rash, so you can compare it to a later date to see if the symptoms have worsened, improved, or stayed the same**

Tracking your symptoms can help you prepare better for any doctor visits.

Possible Causes of an Unhealthy Liver

Although liver damage might be widely associated with excessive alcohol use, an unhealthy liver can also be related to other factors.

Excessive alcohol ingestion

Although it is already a widely known fact that too much alcohol over a prolonged period can cause liver damage, it is still worth noting.

It can be easy to forget the significance of the most widely known things, so it couldn't hurt to serve as a reminder to drink responsibly.

Some people might assume that just because they are not passing out and falling down on the ground, they must not have any problems with alcohol.

"Handling your liquor" does not necessarily mean that the person's liver is handling it well.

Excessive medication usage

Medication, particularly acetaminophen, can be hazardous to the liver when taken in high doses for a prolonged period of time.

Check with a competent doctor about medication usage and follow the instructions on the labels.

Cigarette smoke

Cigarette smoke contains toxic chemicals that the liver has to filter out. This can put a tremendous deal of stress on the liver when high amounts of cigarette smoke are consumed.

Don't forget to stay away from second-hand smoke, as well.

Lack of proper nutrition

The liver is no different from other body organs in the sense that it requires proper nutrition to function at an optimal level.

Poor nutrition can cause liver problems among others.

Even children have been known to have liver problems, and this is suspected to be due to diets that are high in junk food.

Excessive fat from obesity can accumulate around the liver, resulting in fatty liver disease.

Additionally, junk food contains toxins that can place significant stress on the liver, and if it becomes overwhelmed, damage can occur.

Try to keep junk food down to a minimum.

Lack of Sleep

The liver is not immune to the negative effects of sleep deprivation. A lack of sleep can disallow the liver to process fat effectively, which can lead to fatty liver disease.

* * *

If you are curious to know where you stand as far as liver health goes, talk to your doctor about doing a blood test to check your liver enzymes level.

Gallstones

Gallstones are stone-like deposits that form in the gallbladder as a result of hardened bile. They are more common in females than males and are more likely to occur after the age of forty.

They vary in size, ranging from the size of a single grain of sand to as large as a golf ball.

If patients notice signs or symptoms of gallstones, a blood test or ultrasound can confirm whether or not they actually have them.

Symptoms

Many people who have gallstones do not have any noticeable symptoms for years.

Others might get "gallstone attacks" that can come on suddenly and last for up to several hours. These attacks typically include pain in the upper-right portion of the abdomen.

Pain can also occur at the center of the abdomen, the center of the back, and in the right shoulder.

Causes

Possible causes of gallstones are:

- **Ineffective emptying of the gallbladder**
- **Excessive production of a chemical called Bilirubin**
- **Excessive cholesterol in the bile**

Risks

Some of the factors that can put someone at increased risk for gallstones include:

- **Pregnancy**
- **A sedentary lifestyle**
- **Low-fiber diet**
- **High-cholesterol diet**
- **High-fat diet**
- **Diabetes**
- **Losing weight within a very short time period**
- **Obesity**
- **Being over the age of forty**
- **Being female**
- **Liver disease**

- **Having a family history of gallstones**
- **Taking medication that contains estrogen**

Fatty Liver

Fatty Liver Disease is a condition in which the liver has a build up of fat. It can afflict both drinkers and nondrinkers, which splits up the disease into two main groups—Alcoholic Fatty Liver Disease and Nonalcoholic Fatty Liver Disease.

Alcohol Related

If the Fatty Liver Disease is due to excessive alcohol, it falls into the Alcoholic Fatty Liver Disease group.

This is known as the first stage of liver disease that is related to excessive alcohol consumption. If the damage progresses, it can eventually lead to cirrhosis, which is a disease that results in scarring of the liver.

The heavier the person's alcohol consumption, the higher the risk becomes of developing the disease.

A healthy liver does a good job at breaking down much of the alcohol that the person consumes. However, the very process of breaking it down can produce toxic substances that damage liver cells, cause inflammation, and impair the body's natural defense mechanisms.

Nonalcoholic Related

Fatty Liver Disease can also be nonalcoholic related.

If inflammation is minimal to nonexistent, nonalcoholic-related Fatty Liver Disease will generally not cause complications, even if there is fat in the liver.

If there is inflammation in addition to liver cell damage and fat in the liver, fibrosis can result. Fibrosis is a condition that causes scarring of the liver. It can also result in cirrhosis or liver cancer.

Risks

Some of the factors that put a person at risk for Fatty Liver Disease include:

- **Having prediabetes and type 2 diabetes**
- **Having certain metabolic disorders, such as metabolic syndrome**
- **High blood pressure**
- **Being over the age of forty**
- **Obesity**
- **Losing too much weight too rapidly**
- **Exposure to certain toxins**
- **Having certain infections, such as Hepatitis C**

- **Having high cholesterol and triglycerides**
- **Consumption of certain medication**

Diagnosis

Oftentimes, there are no noticeable symptoms for fatty liver, which can make the disease challenging to diagnose.

If a patient with Fatty Liver Disease does have symptoms, they will typically experience discomfort in the upper-right side of the abdomen. The patient might also experience fatigue.

A diagnosis will typically consist of:

- An evaluation of the patient's medical history
- An examination
- Diagnostic imaging tests (X-rays, ultrasound, etc)
- Blood testing
- A biopsy

This doesn't mean you will have to undergo everything in that list. Your doctor might choose to skip the diagnostic imaging and go straight to a blood test after the physical exam.

What to Expect

The doctor will likely ask you:

- If you are currently on any medication
- If you have been consuming any alcohol, and if so, how much and for how long
- If you have any symptoms
- When you started noticing the symptoms

During the physical exam, the doctor will likely press down on different parts of your abdomen, asking you if there is any pain in the area.

At some point, possibly before even seeing the doctor, you might be asked to step on a scale, so they can make a note of your weight. They might also examine your height and check your pulse.

Blood pressure readings are also generally a part of these exams.

The more they know about where you stand medically, the more informed and accurate the diagnosis is likely to be.

While the examination is in progress, the doctor will be searching for signs of an enlarged liver or cirrhosis.

If your doctor decides to put you through diagnostic image testing, he or she will be looking for fat in the liver and stiffness of the liver.

If stiffness in the liver is detected, it can be a sign of liver scarring.

A biopsy may be recommended if liver damage has already been confirmed through blood testing, simply to determine the extent of the liver damage.

It's a good idea to get into the habit of keeping track of medication, symptoms, etc through the use of a journal.

This can help you answer your doctor's questions more accurately.

How to Relieve Liver and Gallbladder Pain Naturally

Although pain relief is not the same thing as curing the underlying cause, some natural remedies can be useful.

Pain relief can cause a person to relax. In return, this relaxation can help the body recuperate and heal itself, depending on what the issue is.

Turmeric

Turmeric is a spice that is known for having anti-inflammatory properties. If the liver or gallbladder pain is caused by inflammation, this spice might be something to try.

Turmeric is commonly found as an ingredient in curry powder. Turmeric powder and curry powder can both be found at many grocery stores in the spices section.

Fresh turmeric is more difficult to find, but some stores may have it.

It has a bitter, peppery taste, so it should be used as part of a recipe for a meal. The rest of the meal will help coat the bitterness.

It can be used in recipes for:

- Soups
- Meat
- Seafood
- Noodles
- Vegetables

Peppermint Tea

Unlike turmeric, peppermint tea doesn't need to be mixed into a recipe, as its taste is refreshing enough to be consumed as a standalone product.

It is caffeine-free, so it can be consumed in the evening without causing trouble in that regard.

It can relieve digestive problems, and since the liver is related to digestion, peppermint tea may provide pain relief.

Additionally, the natural compounds in peppermint can help reduce fatigue and provide energy.

Most grocery stores sell peppermint tea in small boxes that contain peppermint tea bags.

Heat Compress

Applying a heat compress can help relieve pain by getting more blood to flow through the affected area.

While ice is usually recommended for an injury that takes place within forty-eight hours, it is less clear how beneficial it can be for a person who has pain that comes and goes over the course of multiple weeks or months.

For this reason, heat might be a better way to go for the treatment of chronic pain.

Heat can be applied through the use of a heating pad of a hot towel or washcloth, and should not be done for longer than twenty minutes at a time.

Exercise

Exercise has both physical and mental benefits.

The sense of well-being gained from having a good workout can help relieve physical pain.

The movements can also get more blood to flow through the affected area, which can have a similar effect as the heat compress.

* * *

The point of pain relief remedies is to get the body to relax, so that it can effectively heal itself.

But if the symptoms are not going away, the body is probably not healing itself effectively, and additional intervention may be required.

If symptoms continue to return after the remedies, it might be best to see the doctor and get the matter settled.

How to Eliminate Gallstones or Prevent them from Occurring

Whether you already have gallstones or would simply like to prevent them from occurring, the remedies remain essentially the same.

Gold Coin Grass (Lysimachiae herba)

Gold Coin Grass is a herb that grows from a plant.

It is known for its detoxifying qualities, including its ability to treat and prevent cholesterol gallstones.

It also flushes toxins out of the liver.

Lysimachiae herba is available as a supplement that gets distributed:

- in powder form
- in liquid form
- in capsule form
- as extract
- in granule form

It has a sweet, bitter taste, and is generally considered safe to use as long as it is taken in its recommended dosages.

However, since it induces diuresis, this can lead to excessive loss of potassium, which can lead to vertigo if used for an extended period of time.

Other side effects might include allergic reactions, such as contact dermatitis.

Psyllium Husk

Psyllium is a type of fiber that is derived from husks of the Plantago ovata plant's seeds. It is known to defend against the formation of cholesterol gallstones.

To prevent certain types of side effects, it should be taken with plenty of water.

Other side effects include allergic reactions, such as anaphylaxis, which can be fatal.

It is often distributed in powder form and can be purchased online.

*　*　*

If you have gallstones and neither of these products rectify the issue, surgery may be necessary.

How to Reverse Fatty Liver

Generally, Fatty Liver Disease is only reversible when it is in its initial stage, referred to as, Nonalcoholic Fatty Liver.

If it progresses to Nonalcoholic Steatohepatitis, the damage may be irreversible. That's why it's important not to wait too long before getting a diagnosis and receiving treatment.

Weight Loss

If you are in the initial stage of Fatty Liver Disease, and are overweight, weight loss is critical.

One of the good things about weight loss is that you don't have to starve. In fact, eating more frequently will speed up the metabolism.

Of course, you still have to eat the right foods and in the right amounts.

Aim for 6-8 small meals a day, spread out over the course of every two hours.

Cut out the junk food and focus on quality food products.

Quality food products that can leave you with a feeling of fullness include:

- Oatmeal
- Eggs
- Whole-grain bagels
- Whole-grain pasta
- Baked potatoes
- Lean meat
- Brown rice

Even though fruits and vegetables might not be very filling, it's important to include them as part of a healthy diet.

Use healthy fats, such as olive oil and fatty fish.

Remember, toxins place stress on the liver. Try to stick with organic products as often as possible.

The portions should be small. To help yourself feel more full, consume each meal with two glasses of water, preferably cold water.

Drinking cold beverages can help burn extra calories.

It's also important to keep track of how many calories you are consuming. It makes no sense to increase meal frequency to speed up the metabolism if you are consuming twice the amount of calories you were before you started the new diet.

In addition to consuming healthy foods more frequently, reduce your daily allotment of calories by approximately five hundred.

Try to exercise regularly. Half an hour to forty-five minutes of cardio five times a week should be adequate.

Omega-3 Fatty Acids

Along with many other health benefits, Omega-3 fatty acids have been known to reduce liver fat. Try to include Omega-3 fatty acids in your diet most of the days of the week.

Omega-3 fat can be found in fatty fish, such as salmon.

Avoid fish that have high mercury content.

Here are two lists that separate fish with high and low levels of mercury:

High Levels of Mercury

- Orange roughy
- Halibut
- Swordfish
- Shark
- King mackerel
- Gulf tilefish
- Marlin
- Grouper
- Tuna (light tuna is considered somewhat lower in mercury than albacore)
- Spanish mackerel
- Sablefish
- Bluefish
- Chilean

Low Levels of Mercury

- Atlantic mackerel
- Cat fish
- Crab
- Crawfish
- Haddock
- Oysters
- Sardines
- Scallops
- Shrimp
- Squid
- Tilapia
- Trout

- Wild and Alaska salmon

You might also want to take a fish oil supplement. Try to find one that states on the label that it does not contain mercury.

Green Tea

Green tea contains antioxidants that help reduce liver fat and inflammation. The product can be found in most grocery stores and typically comes in small boxes that contain green tea bags.

Soluble Fiber

Soluble fiber can help decrease liver fat. Additionally, it can help lower liver enzyme levels and increase insulin sensitivity.

Aim for approximately 10 grams of soluble fiber a day.

Foods that contain soluble fiber include:

- Apricots
- Apples
- Avocados
- Black beans
- Broccoli
- Carrots
- Figs
- Flaxseeds
- Nectarines
- Oats
- Sunflower seeds
- Sweet potatoes

Whey Protein

Whey is a type of protein that can decrease liver fat and lower liver enzyme levels.

Whey protein powder can be found at health supplement stores and in certain grocery stores.

To make a liver-healthy whey protein drink, blend:

- 1 serving of whey protein powder
- 8-12 oz of milk
- 2-3 tablespoons of olive oil

Chocolate-flavored protein powder is recommended, so when it's mixed with milk, it will taste like chocolate milk.

You can also experiment with different combinations, such as plain water mixed with protein powder and possibly a little bit of honey for flavor.

Personally, I had actually regularly blended chocolate protein powder with orange juice in the past, and it turned out well.

But everyone will have their own set of likes and dislikes, so keep experimenting until you find a favorable recipe.

How to Diet After Gallbladder Removal

Patients who choose to have their gallbladder removed will generally need to undergo a change in their diet.

Since the gallbladder helps digest foods that have high-fat content, it is typically good to avoid fatty foods within the first few days after surgery.

During the first few days after surgery, it is better to stick with very light foods that are easy to digest.

These light foods can include:

- Jello
- Broth
- Clear liquids

After the first few days are over, solid foods can be introduced into the diet, but they should be kept light.

Light solid food can include:

- Toast
- Crackers (preferably unsalted)
- Plain noodles
- Plain rice
- Dry cereal

Exactly how long each person should stay on the light solid food diet is not entirely clear, since different people can have different reactions.

But typically, the light solid food diet should only need to be followed for the first few weeks after surgery, although some patients still have trouble digesting spicy foods a few months after gallbladder removal.

Introduce heavier foods very gradually, and see what the response is. If a heavier dish causes pain or digestive issues, it is best to go back to consuming lighter foods. Then try reintroducing heavier foods at at later time.

Keep meals small and frequent, and keep a journal of which foods seem to bother you the most.

It can also help to have an appetizer before a meal. This is especially useful if you plan on having a heavier dish.

Having greasy food on an empty stomach is more likely to cause problems than greasy food on a partially full stomach.

If you plan on having meat for dinner, try starting the meal with vegetables first. Then have some soup before consuming the meat.

If problems still occur, even after "warming up" with the appetizers, the "problem foods" will need to be eliminated, at least for a while.

Try to keep your daily fat intake under 30% of your daily overall calorie consumption.

Closing

Although certain health problems can seem overwhelming, they shouldn't be feared. They should simply be seen as problems that need to be corrected.

Most medical problems are fixable, or at least treatable, and many of them only require minor lifestyle changes.

If liver and gallbladder issues are found early enough, it is often only a matter simple lifestyle changes to correct the problems.

Diet plays a large role. By consuming the right diet for your particular situation, symptoms can be cured, or at least managed, effectively.

Exercise is also important, as it can relieve pain, boost moods, and burn excess calories.

Staying healthy is not only beneficial for the liver and gallbladder, but for all other body organs as well.

www.ingramcontent.com/pod-product-compliance
Lightning Source LLC
Chambersburg PA
CBHW080821220526
45466CB00011BB/3642